# "THE JOURNEY TO WELLNESS: 10 DIETS FOR A HEALTHIER AND LIGHTER LIFE"

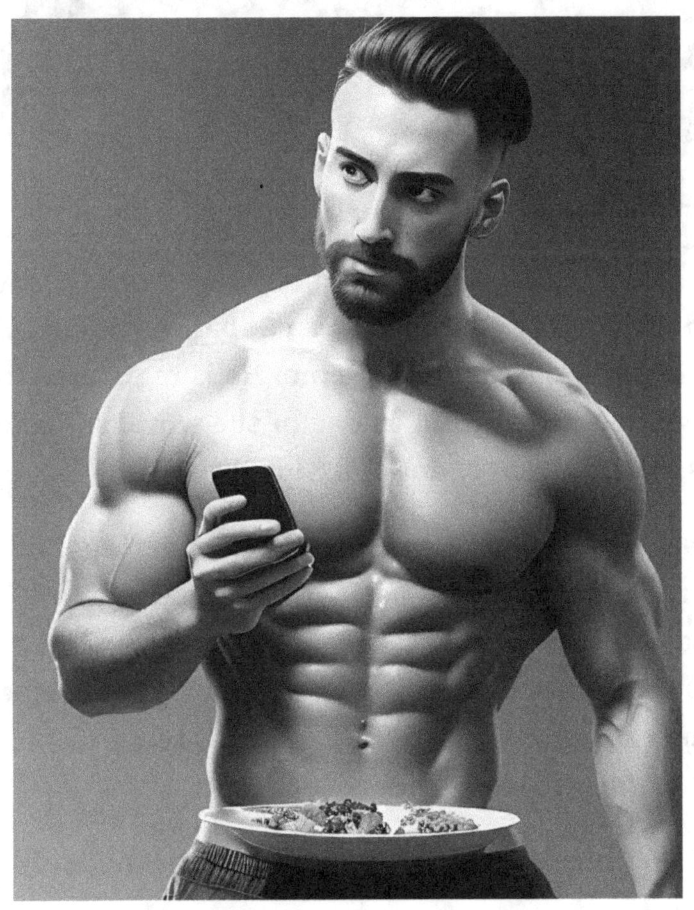

# **<u>Author:</u>**

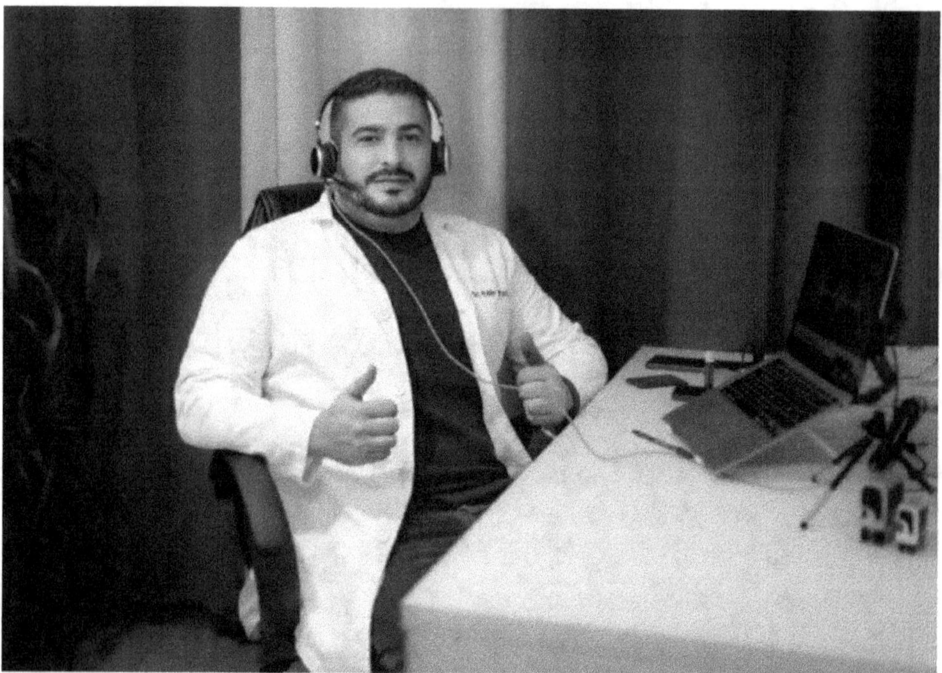

**Dr. Pablo Odeley Puente Fumero is a Cuban-American physician specializing in Emergency Medicine. He is registered in Madrid and has gained recognition as one of the world's top doctors in 2022, selected by Top100doc and Global Submit.**

**Dr. Puente Fumero is committed to delivering high-quality healthcare and ensuring patient safety. He stays updated on the latest advancements in Emergency Medicine through continuous education and professional development. His dedication to his field is exemplified by his recognition as one of the top 100 doctors worldwide.**

**Beyond his clinical work, Dr. Puente Fumero is actively involved**

in medical research and contributes to the advancement of knowledge in Emergency Medicine. He believes in the importance of evidence-based medicine and utilizes the latest research findings to inform his practice.

With his expertise, dedication, and recognition as a top doctor, Dr. Pablo Odeley Puente Fumero serves as an invaluable asset to the medical community. His commitment to providing excellent emergency care and his contributions to medical research make him a respected and trusted physician in his field.

More in: www.medico.red

**Table of Contents**

## Introduction

Welcome to "The Journey to Wellness: 10 Diets for a Healthier and Lighter Life". This book is a practical guide designed to help you navigate the world of weight loss diets, providing you with the information you need to make informed decisions about the best diet for you. Weight loss and proper nutrition are essential elements of overall health and well-being. This book was created with the goal of providing a variety of diets and meal plans to help you achieve your weight loss goals in a healthy and sustainable manner. Each of us is unique, and what works for one may not work for another. Therefore, we have compiled a variety of diets, each with its own approach and philosophy on weight loss and nutrition. From green detox to intermittent fasting and the Mediterranean diet, there's something for everyone. In each chapter, we'll introduce a different diet, explaining its basic principles, potential benefits, and the challenges you might face while following that plan. We'll also provide you with a 7-day meal outline as a sample for each diet. Always speak with a healthcare professional. Make sure the plan you choose is suitable for your specific health needs and lifestyle. Nutrition is a complex science and each individual has unique needs.

Remember, this book is not only about weight loss. It's also about building a sustainable lifestyle that allows you to feel better and live more fully.

We hope this book serves as a helpful resource on your journey to health and wellness. Let's embark on this journey together towards a healthier, lighter life!

Note for all chapters: Be sure to consult a doctor or a nutritionist before starting the plan. Portions and variety of foods can vary based on individual needs.

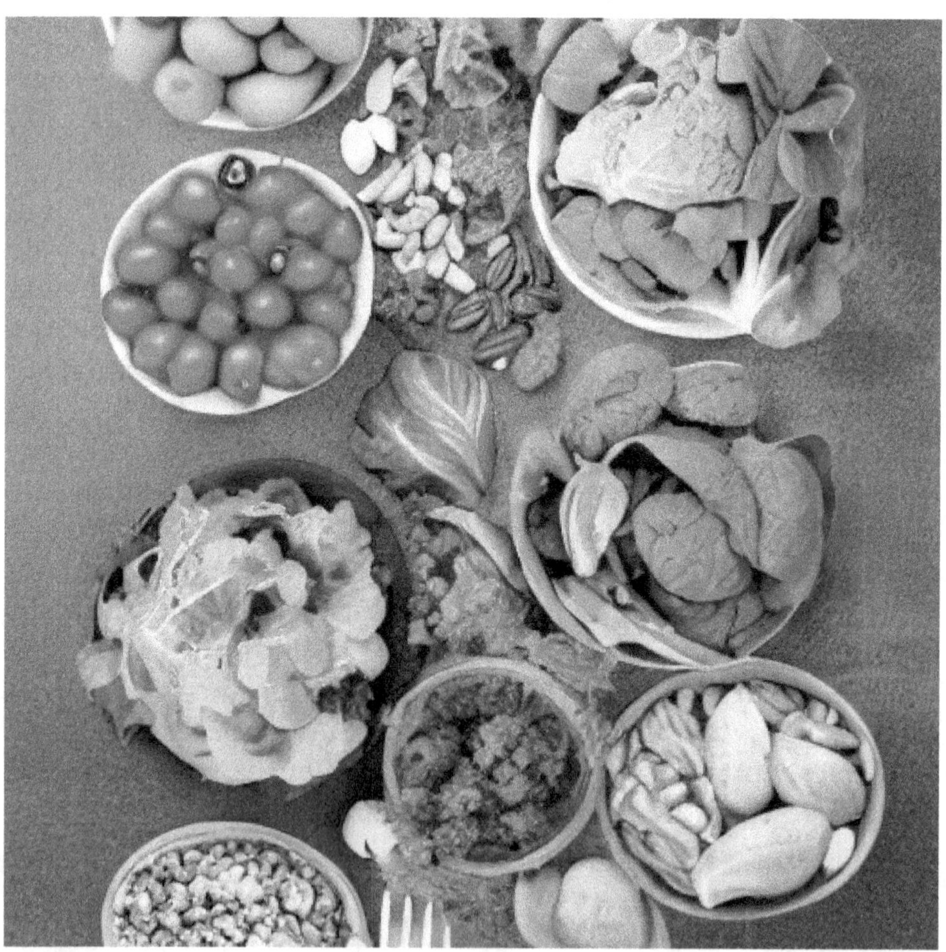

## Chapter 1: Green Detox Diet

Introduction to the Green Detox Diet

The Green Detox Diet centers on the idea of cleansing and rejuvenating the body by incorporating nutrient-rich foods and eliminating toxins. This meal plan emphasizes leafy green vegetables, fruits, nuts, seeds, and whole grains. Through this approach, the aim is to boost energy, improve digestion, and promote healthy weight loss.

Benefits and Challenges

Benefits:

• Increase in nutrient intake, such as vitamins, minerals, and antioxidants.

• Improved digestion and liver function.

• Promotes weight loss by reducing the consumption of processed and high-calorie foods.

• Encourages proper hydration through the consumption of juices and smoothies.

Challenges:

• It can be difficult to follow in the long term due to the restriction of certain food groups.

• Possible fatigue and weakness at the start of the diet due to a reduction in calorie intake.

• Preparing juices and smoothies can require time and specialized equipment.

7-Day Meal Plan

Note: Be sure to consult a doctor or a nutritionist before starting the plan. Portions and variety of foods can vary based on individual needs.

Day 1

• Breakfast: Green smoothie (spinach, kale, pineapple, green apple, coconut water)

• Lunch: Spinach salad with lemon and avocado dressing, nuts, and pepitas

• Dinner: Broccoli and spinach soup with chunks of avocado
• Snacks: Carrots and hummus; handful of almonds
Day 2
• Breakfast: Berry and spinach smoothie (strawberries, blueberries, spinach, coconut water)
• Lunch: Quinoa salad and vegetables with honey mustard dressing
• Dinner: Steamed asparagus with lemon sauce and almonds
• Snacks: Cucumber slices and hummus; handful of cashews
Day 3
• Breakfast: Kale, banana, and almond butter smoothie
• Lunch: Lettuce wrap filled with avocado, tomato, and cucumber
• Dinner: Cauliflower puree with garlic mushrooms
• Snacks: Celery and peanut butter; handful of pistachios
Day 4
• Breakfast: Pineapple, mango, and spinach smoothie
• Lunch: Chickpea and vegetable salad with lemon and olive oil dressing
• Dinner: Zucchini spaghetti with tomato and basil sauce
• Snacks: Bell peppers
Day 5
• Breakfast: Spinach, green apple, and chia seeds smoothie
• Lunch: Quinoa bowl with broccoli, carrots, bell peppers, and low-sodium soy sauce
• Dinner: Lentil soup with vegetables and spices
• Snacks: Carrot sticks and hummus; handful of walnuts
Day 6
• Breakfast: Kale, blueberry, and flaxseed smoothie
• Lunch: Spinach salad with walnuts, strawberries, and balsamic dressing
• Dinner: Oven-baked zucchini stuffed with quinoa and vegetables
• Snacks: Celery and almond butter; handful of pumpkin seeds
Day 7
• Breakfast: Spinach, banana, and peanut butter smoothie
• Lunch: Brown rice bowl with tofu, broccoli, carrots, and teriyaki sauce

• Dinner: Homemade tomato soup with toasted whole grain bread
• Snacks: Cucumber slices and guacamole; handful of almonds
Remember, the Green Detox Diet is an excellent way to increase your nutrient intake and cleanse your system, but it's important to consider your individual nutritional needs. If you feel hungry, don't hesitate to add more fruits, vegetables, whole grains, and plant proteins to your day. The key is to listen to your body and nourish it with quality foods.

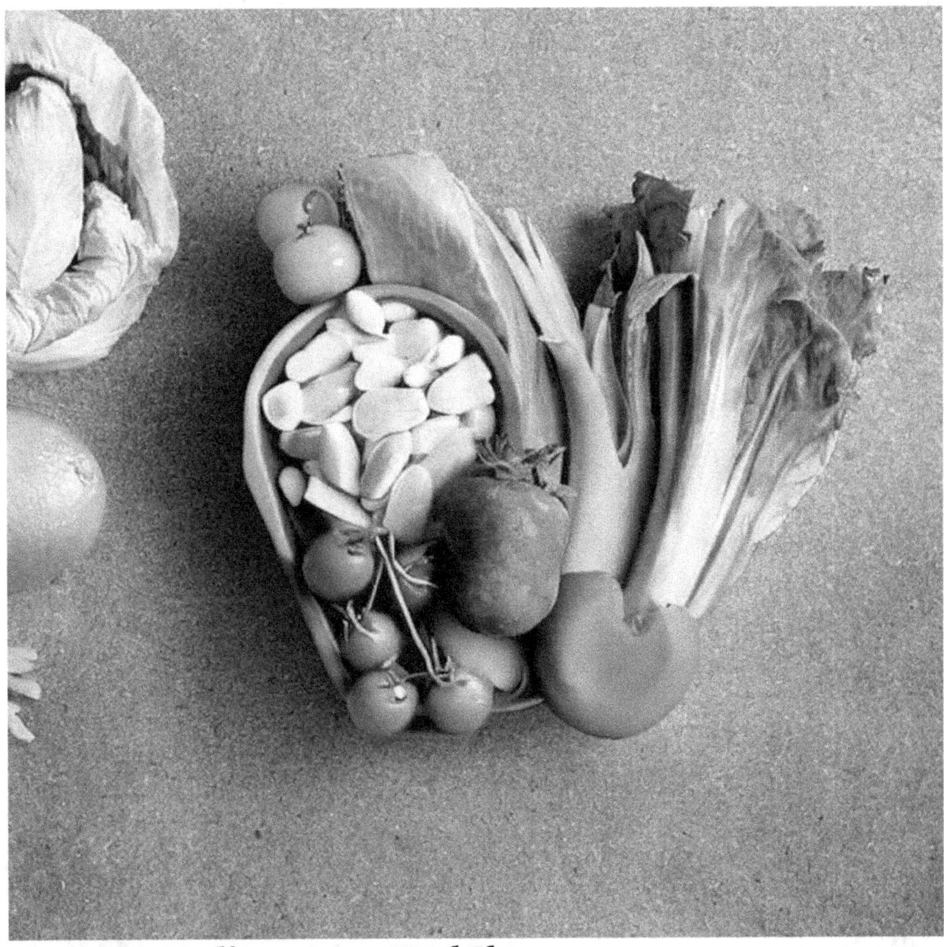

## Chapter 2: Mediterranean Meal Plan

Introduction to the Mediterranean Meal Plan

The Mediterranean Meal Plan is based on the traditional eating habits of people living in countries bordering the Mediterranean Sea, such as Italy, Greece, Spain, and Morocco. This diet emphasizes whole, fresh, and seasonal foods, and includes a significant number of fruits, vegetables, whole grains, legumes, olive oil, nuts, and seeds, with moderation in fish, dairy, and wine, and limiting red meat and processed foods.

Benefits and Challenges
Benefits:
• Widely recognized for its heart health benefits.
• Rich in essential nutrients, including fiber, protein, healthy fats, and antioxidants.
• Promotes weight loss by focusing on high-quality and nutritious foods.
• Encourages mindful eating and enjoying meals with others.
Challenges:
• May require more time for cooking and food preparation.
• Fresh, high-quality foods can be more expensive.
• Can be a significant change for those accustomed to diets high in red meat and processed foods.

7-Day Meal Plan
Note: Be sure to speak with a health professional before starting this meal plan or any other. Portions and variety of foods may vary depending on individual needs.
Day 1
• Breakfast: Whole grain toast with avocado and tomato
• Lunch: Greek salad with olives, feta cheese, olive oil, and lemon dressing
• Dinner: Baked salmon with quinoa and roasted vegetables
• Snacks: Almonds; Greek yogurt with honey and walnuts
Day 2
• Breakfast: Homemade granola with Greek yogurt and berries

- Lunch: Lentil soup with whole grain bread
- Dinner: Grilled chicken with couscous salad
- Snacks: Hummus with carrots; handful of pistachios

Day 3

- Breakfast: Fruit smoothie with spinach and chia seeds
- Lunch: Quinoa bowl with chickpeas, tomato, cucumber, and tahini dressing
- Dinner: Grilled white fish with potato salad
- Snacks: Feta cheese with olives; Greek yogurt with pomegranate

Day 4

- Breakfast: Whole grain toast with olive oil, tomato, and feta cheese
- Lunch: Tomato and basil soup with whole grain bread
- Dinner: Whole grain pasta with tomato sauce, garlic, capers, and anchovies
- Snacks: Dried fruits; Greek yogurt with honey

Day 5

- Breakfast: Fruit salad with Greek yogurt and a handful of almonds
- Lunch: Tuna and tomato salad, olives and olive oil, and lemon dressing
- Dinner: Stewed lentils with vegetables and whole grain bread
- Snacks: Feta cheese and grapes; a handful of nuts

Day 6

- Breakfast: Whole grain toast with almond butter and banana slices
- Lunch: Chickpea salad with cucumber, tomato, bell pepper, and tahini dressing
- Dinner: Grilled fish with baked potatoes and spinach salad
- Snacks: Hummus with carrots; Greek yogurt with honey and walnuts

Day 7

- Breakfast: Fruit smoothie with Greek yogurt and chia seeds
- Lunch: Tabbouleh with whole grain pita bread

- Dinner: Grilled chicken with quinoa salad and roasted vegetables
- Snacks: Olives and feta cheese; a handful of almonds

The Mediterranean Meal Plan is not just a diet, but a lifestyle that emphasizes the quality of food, mindful eating, and enjoyment of meals with family and friends. Remember, it's important to adapt any meal plan to your individual needs and preferences.

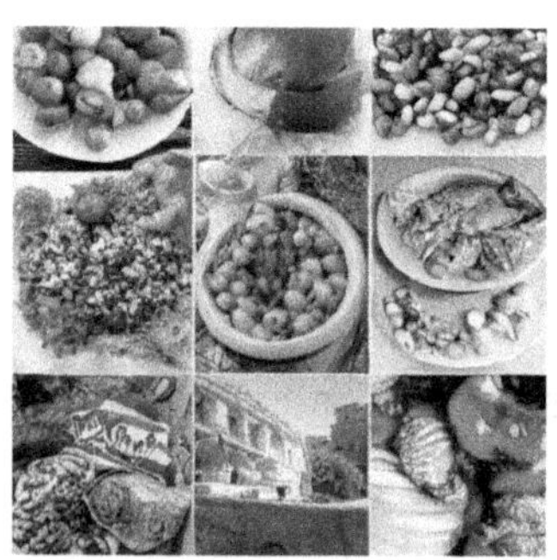

## Chapter 3: The 5-Ingredient Diet

Introduction to the 5-Ingredient Diet

The 5-Ingredient Diet is an approach to eating that focuses on simplifying meals and ingredients. The idea is to make each meal using five ingredients or less, not including basic seasonings like salt, pepper, and olive oil. This approach can help eliminate processed foods and promote the use of whole, high-quality foods.

Benefits and Challenges

Benefits:
- Simplifies meal planning.
- Can help reduce the intake of processed foods and increase the

consumption of whole foods.
- Can help improve awareness and appreciation of each ingredient.

Challenges:
- May require more time and effort in the kitchen.
- May limit the variety of meals if not creative.
- Some healthy and nutritious meals may require more than five ingredients.

7-Day Meal Plan

Note: Be sure to consult a healthcare professional before starting this or any other meal plan. Portion sizes and food variety may vary based on individual needs.

Day 1
- Breakfast: Banana, spinach, almond butter, almond milk, and chia smoothie.
- Lunch: Grilled chicken salad with spinach, strawberries, walnuts, and olive oil dressing.
- Dinner: Baked salmon, quinoa, and steamed broccoli.
- Snack: Apple and almond butter.

Day 2
- Breakfast: Scrambled eggs with spinach and feta cheese.
- Lunch: Chickpea salad with cucumber, tomato, parsley, and olive oil dressing.
- Dinner: Baked chicken breast, roasted sweet potatoes, and green salad.
- Snack: Greek yogurt, honey, and nuts.

Day 3
- Breakfast: Oatmeal with apple, cinnamon, honey, and nuts.
- Lunch: Tuna salad with lettuce, tomato, cucumber, and olive oil.
- Dinner: Grilled white fish, quinoa, and steamed asparagus.
- Snack: Carrots and hummus.

Day 4
- Breakfast: Whole wheat toast with avocado and poached egg.

- Lunch: Grilled chicken salad with quinoa, tomato, cucumber, and olive oil dressing.
- Dinner: Grilled steak, baked potatoes, and green salad.
- Snack: Greek yogurt, honey, and berries.

Day 5
- Breakfast: Mixed berry smoothie with Greek yogurt, honey, and chia seeds.
- Lunch: Grilled salmon salad with spinach, tomato, walnuts, and olive oil dressing.
- Dinner: Grilled chicken breast, quinoa, and steamed broccoli.
- Snack: Apple and almond butter.

Day 6
- Breakfast: Whole wheat toast with avocado and tomato.
- Lunch: Chickpea salad with spinach, feta cheese, cucumber, and olive oil dressing.
- Dinner: Baked fish fillet, roasted potatoes, and green salad.
- Snack: Greek yogurt, honey, and nuts.

Day 7
- Breakfast: Oatmeal with banana, almond butter, and honey.
- Lunch: Grilled chicken salad with spinach, quinoa, walnuts, and olive oil dressing.
- Dinner: Baked salmon, roasted sweet potatoes, and steamed asparagus.
- Snack: Carrots and hummus.

The 5-Ingredient Diet can be an excellent way to simplify meals and focus on whole, nutritious foods. However, it's important to remember that variety is key to a healthy diet, so it's essential to be creative and experiment with different food combinations to ensure a complete range of nutrients.

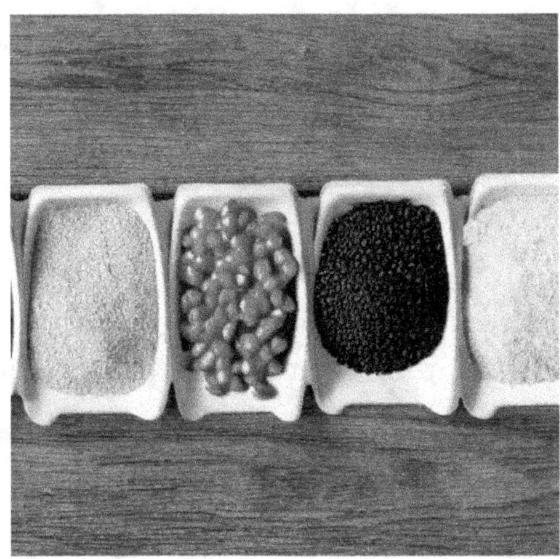

## Chapter 4: Intermittent Fasting Diet

Introduction to Intermittent Fasting

Intermittent fasting is an eating approach that alternates between periods of eating and fasting. It doesn't focus so much on what foods you should eat but rather when you should eat them. There are several methods of intermittent fasting, but the most common ones include the 16/8 method (fasting for 16 hours, with an 8-hour feeding window), the 5:2 method (eating normally for 5 days, reducing calorie intake to 500-600 on 2 non-consecutive days), and the eat-stop-eat method (complete fasting for 24 hours once or twice a week).

Benefits and Challenges

Benefits:
- Can promote weight loss and significantly improve insulin sensitivity.
- Can help simplify meal schedules and reduce meal planning-related stress.
- Some research suggests benefits for heart and brain health.

Challenges:
- May be difficult to follow, especially at the beginning.

- Not suitable for everyone, especially those with certain medical conditions or a history of eating disorders.
- May lead to overeating or unhealthy eating during feeding windows.

7-Day Meal Plan (16/8 Method)

Note: Be sure to consult a healthcare professional before starting this or any other meal plan. Portion sizes and food variety may vary based on individual needs.

For this plan, a feeding window from 12 pm to 8 pm was chosen. During fasting hours, you can drink water, tea, and coffee without sugar.

Day 1
- 12 pm: Grilled chicken salad with olive oil dressing.
- 3 pm: Handful of almonds and an apple.
- 6 pm: Baked salmon with quinoa and steamed broccoli.
- 8 pm: Greek yogurt with honey and nuts.

Day 2
- 12 pm: Avocado toast with scrambled eggs.
- 3 pm: Carrots and hummus.
- 6 pm: Grilled chicken with couscous salad.
- 8 pm: One cup of strawberries and an ounce of dark chocolate.

Day 3
- 12 pm: Quinoa bowl with grilled vegetables and tofu.
- 3 pm: Apple and almond butter.
- 6 pm: Grilled white fish with mashed sweet potatoes and steamed asparagus.
- 8 pm: Greek yogurt with homemade granola.

Day 4
- 12 pm: Tuna salad with olive oil and lemon.
- 3 pm: Cucumber and hummus.
- 6 pm: Baked chicken breast with roasted potatoes and green salad.

- 8 pm: One cup of mixed berries with a handful of almonds.

Day 5
- 12 pm: Quinoa salad with fresh vegetables and lemon olive oil dressing.
- 3 pm: Handful of nuts and a pear.
- 6 pm: Grilled salmon with spinach salad and balsamic vinegar dressing.
- 8 pm: Greek yogurt with a drizzle of honey and chopped nuts.

Day 6
- 12 pm: Scrambled eggs with spinach and feta cheese, served on whole wheat toast.
- 3 pm: Carrots and hummus.
- 6 pm: Grilled chicken breast with quinoa and steamed broccoli.
- 8 pm: One cup of fresh pineapple and a handful of almonds.

Day 7
- 12 pm: Chickpea salad with tomatoes, cucumbers, peppers, and tahini dressing.
- 3 pm: Apple and almond butter.
- 6 pm: Grilled white fish with mashed sweet potatoes and steamed asparagus.
- 8 pm: One cup of strawberries with a drizzle of melted dark chocolate.

Intermittent fasting can be a useful tool for weight loss and health management, but it's important to remember that the quality of the foods you consume during your feeding windows is equally important. Choose nutritious and balanced foods to ensure your body gets the nutrients it needs to function optimally.

## Chapter 5: Whole Food Plant-Based Diet

Introduction to the Whole Food Plant-Based Diet

The Whole Food Plant-Based Diet focuses on consuming foods in their most natural or minimally processed form. It includes fruits, vegetables, legumes, whole grains, nuts, and seeds, while avoiding animal products and processed foods. It's not necessarily a vegetarian or vegan diet, but it prioritizes plant-based foods.

Benefits and Challenges

Benefits:
- Can help prevent and treat chronic diseases such as heart disease, diabetes, and obesity.
- Is sustainable and environmentally friendly.
- Promotes variety and the intake of a wide range of nutrients.

Challenges:
- May require more time and effort in meal preparation.
- Can be challenging to follow when eating out or in social situations.
- May require supplementation of certain nutrients, such as vitamin B12.

7-Day Meal Plan

Note: Be sure to consult a healthcare professional before starting this or any other meal plan. Portion sizes and food variety may vary based on individual needs.

Day 1
- Breakfast: Oatmeal with mixed berries, chia seeds, and nuts.
- Lunch: Quinoa salad with cucumber, tomato, bell peppers, chickpeas, and olive oil and lemon dressing.
- Dinner: Lentil curry with brown rice.
- Snack: Apple and almond butter.

Day 2

- Breakfast: Spinach, banana, almond butter, almond milk, and chia seed smoothie.
- Lunch: Chickpea salad with spinach, tomato, cucumber, and tahini dressing.
- Dinner: Grilled tofu with quinoa and steamed broccoli.
- Snack: Carrots and hummus.

Day 3
- Breakfast: Whole wheat toast with avocado and chia seeds.
- Lunch: Lentil salad with spinach, carrot, bell pepper, and olive oil and lemon dressing.
- Dinner: Quinoa and black bean stuffed peppers, served with a green salad.
- Snack: Mixed berries and soy yogurt.

Day 4
- Breakfast: Mixed berry, soy milk, flax seeds, and spinach smoothie.
- Lunch: Quinoa salad with cherry tomatoes, cucumber, olives, olive oil, and balsamic vinegar.
- Dinner: Lentil stew with whole wheat bread.
- Snack: Nuts and a pear.

Day 5
- Breakfast: Oatmeal with banana, nuts, and chia seeds.
- Lunch: Hummus with raw vegetables for dipping and whole wheat pita bread.
- Dinner: Whole wheat pasta with homemade tomato sauce and a green salad.
- Snack: Soy yogurt with mixed berries.

Day 6
- Breakfast: Whole wheat toast with almond butter and banana.
- Lunch: Black bean salad with corn, tomato, avocado, and olive oil and lime dressing.
- Dinner: Baked tofu with roasted sweet potatoes and steamed asparagus.

- Snack: Carrots and hummus.

Day 7
- Breakfast: Banana, spinach, chia seeds, and almond milk smoothie.
- Lunch: Chickpea salad with cucumber, tomato, bell pepper, and tahini dressing.
- Dinner: Quinoa and black bean stuffed peppers, served with a green salad.
- Snack: Apple and almond butter.

The Whole Food Plant-Based Diet can be an excellent way to improve health and support a sustainable lifestyle. However, it's important to remember that variety and the quality of foods are key to ensuring a complete range of nutrients. It can be helpful to work with a dietitian or healthcare professional to ensure all nutritional needs are adequately met.

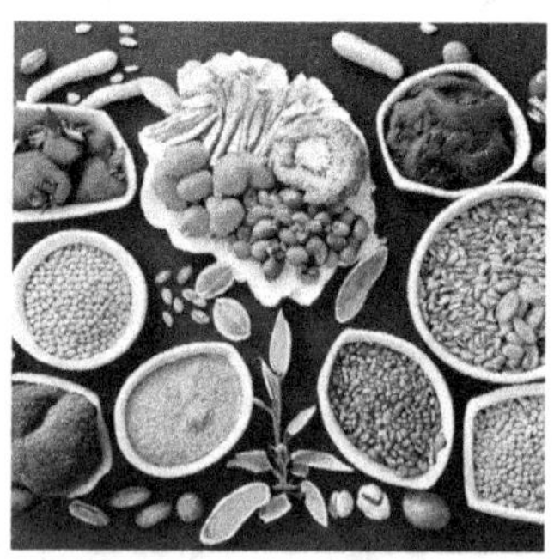

## Chapter 6: Lean Protein and Vegetable Diet

Introduction to the Lean Protein and Vegetable Diet

The Lean Protein and Vegetable Diet is an eating approach that prioritizes high-quality proteins and vegetables while minimizing processed carbohydrates and sugars. Protein sources can include lean meats, fish, eggs, tofu, and legumes, while vegetables can be of any type, preferably leafy greens and a variety of colors to ensure a wide range of nutrients.

Benefits and Challenges

Benefits:
- Can aid in weight loss by promoting satiety and reducing calorie intake.
- Can improve blood sugar control and reduce the risk of cardiovascular and chronic diseases.
- Promotes the intake of a wide range of nutrients through a variety of vegetables.

Challenges:
- May require more time and effort in meal preparation.
- Can be challenging to follow when eating out or in social situations.
- Reducing carbohydrates may be difficult for some individuals, especially at the beginning.

7-Day Meal Plan

Note: Be sure to consult a healthcare professional before starting this or any other meal plan. Portion sizes and food variety may vary based on individual needs.

Day 1
- Breakfast: Scrambled eggs with spinach and tomato.
- Lunch: Grilled chicken salad with lettuce, cucumber, bell pepper, and olive oil and lemon dressing.
- Dinner: Baked salmon with steamed broccoli and quinoa.
- Snack: Carrots and hummus.

Day 2
- Breakfast: Protein smoothie with spinach, banana, and almond butter.
- Lunch: Tuna salad with lettuce, tomato, cucumber, and olive oil and balsamic vinegar dressing.
- Dinner: Grilled chicken breast with quinoa salad and roasted vegetables.
- Snack: Greek yogurt with mixed berries.

Day 3
- Breakfast: Whole wheat toast with avocado and poached egg.
- Lunch: Chickpea salad with spinach, cucumber, bell pepper, and olive oil and lemon dressing.
- Dinner: Grilled beef steak with baked potatoes and steamed asparagus.
- Snack: Apple and almond butter.

Day 4
- Breakfast: Protein smoothie with mixed berries, spinach, and chia seeds.
- Lunch: Grilled chicken salad with lettuce, tomato, carrot, and olive oil and balsamic vinegar dressing.
- Dinner: Baked white fish with quinoa and roasted vegetables.
- Snack: Greek yogurt with almonds.

Day 5
- Breakfast: Scrambled eggs with spinach and mushrooms.
- Lunch: Chickpea salad with spinach, cucumber, tomato, and tahini dressing.
- Dinner: Grilled chicken breast with green salad and roasted sweet potatoes.
- Snack: Carrots and hummus.

Day 6
- Breakfast: Whole wheat toast with avocado and poached egg.
- Lunch: Tuna salad with lettuce, tomato, cucumber, and olive oil and lemon dressing.
- Dinner: Baked salmon with steamed broccoli and quinoa.
- Snack: Apple and almond butter.

Day 7
- Breakfast: Protein smoothie with banana, spinach, and almond butter.
- Lunch: Grilled chicken salad with lettuce, cucumber, carrot, and olive oil and balsamic vinegar dressing.
- Dinner: Grilled beef steak with baked potatoes and steamed

asparagus.
- Snack: Greek yogurt with mixed berries.

The Lean Protein and Vegetable Diet can be an excellent way to improve health, lose weight, and maintain muscle. However, it's important to remember that variety and the quality of foods are key to ensuring a complete range of nutrients. It can be helpful to work with a dietitian or healthcare professional to ensure all nutritional needs are adequately met.

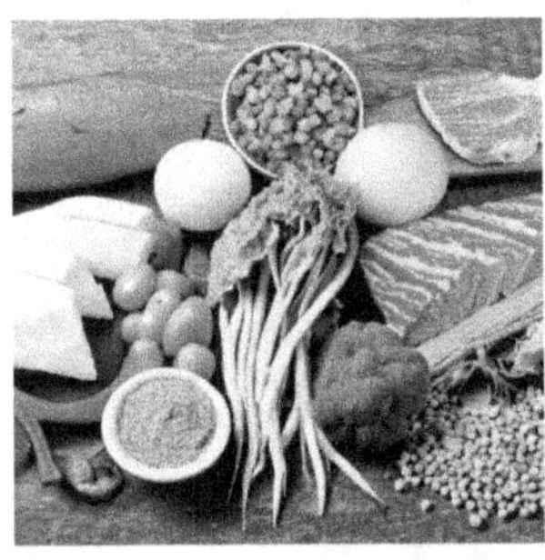

## Chapter 7: Flexitarian Meal Plan

Introduction to the Flexitarian Diet

The flexitarian diet, a term combining "flexible" and "vegetarian," was created by dietitian Dawn Jackson Blatner. This diet is primarily plant-based but allows for moderate consumption of meat and other animal products. It is more of a lifestyle than a strict diet, as there are no rigid rules or prohibitions, but it encourages choosing healthier and more sustainable foods.

Benefits and Challenges

Benefits:
- Can aid in weight loss and improve health.
- Reduces carbon footprint and is more environmentally friendly.
- Offers flexibility and may be easier to follow long-term than strictly vegetarian or vegan diets.

Challenges:
- May require more time and effort in meal preparation.
- Can be challenging to follow when eating out or in social situations.

7-Day Meal Plan

Note: Be sure to consult a healthcare professional before starting this or any other meal plan. Portion sizes and food variety may vary based on individual needs.

Day 1
- Breakfast: Oatmeal with mixed berries and nuts.
- Lunch: Quinoa salad with roasted vegetables and hummus.
- Dinner: Grilled fish with steamed asparagus and baked potatoes.
- Snack: Apple with almond butter.

Day 2
- Breakfast: Spinach, banana, and almond butter smoothie.
- Lunch: Lentil salad with raw vegetables and olive oil and balsamic vinegar dressing.
- Dinner: Grilled tofu with quinoa and steamed broccoli.
- Snack: Greek yogurt with mixed berries.

Day 3
- Breakfast: Whole wheat toast with avocado and chia seeds.
- Lunch: Vegetable soup with a handful of chickpeas.
- Dinner: Grilled chicken with green salad and baked sweet potatoes.
- Snack: Carrots and hummus.

Day 4
- Breakfast: Protein smoothie with spinach, mixed berries, and flax seeds.
- Lunch: Chickpea salad with spinach, cucumber, tomato, and tahini dressing.
- Dinner: Baked white fish with quinoa and roasted vegetables.
- Snack: Greek yogurt with almonds.

Day 5
- Breakfast: Oatmeal with banana, nuts, and chia seeds.
- Lunch: Quinoa salad with roasted vegetables and hummus.
- Dinner: Grilled chicken with green salad and baked potatoes.
- Snack: Apple with almond butter.

Day 6

- Breakfast: Whole wheat toast with avocado and chia seeds.
- Lunch: Vegetable soup with a handful of lentils.
- Dinner: Grilled tofu with quinoa and steamed broccoli.
- Snack: Greek yogurt with mixed berries.

Day 7
- Breakfast: Protein smoothie with banana, spinach, and almond butter.
- Lunch: Chickpea salad with spinach, cucumber, tomato, and tahini dressing.
- Dinner: Grilled chicken with green salad and baked sweet potatoes.
- Snack: Carrots and hummus.

The Flexitarian Diet can be an excellent way to improve health, reduce environmental impact, and maintain a balanced and nutritious diet. However, it's important to remember that variety and the quality of foods are key to ensuring a complete range of nutrients. It can be helpful to work with a dietitian or healthcare professional to ensure all nutritional needs are adequately met.

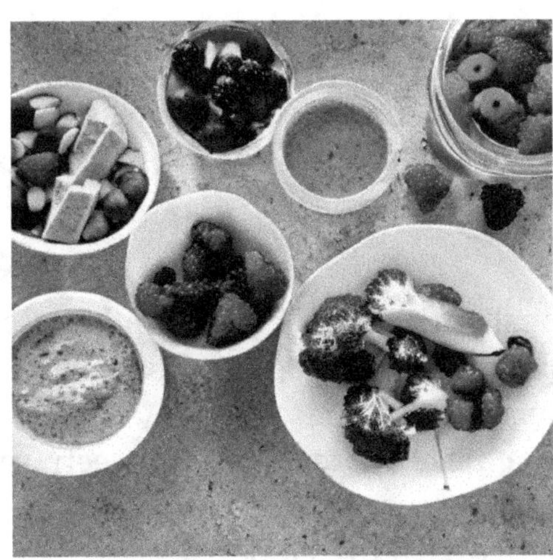

## Chapter 8: DASH Diet (Dietary Approaches to Stop Hypertension)

## Introduction to the DASH Diet

The DASH Diet is a meal plan specifically developed to help improve blood pressure. DASH stands for "Dietary Approaches to Stop Hypertension." This eating plan focuses on fruits, vegetables, whole grains, and lean meats.

## Benefits and Challenges

Benefits:
- Proven to lower blood pressure and reduce the risk of heart disease.
- Can aid in weight loss.
- Encourages the intake of a variety of nutrient-rich foods.

Challenges:
- May require more time and effort in meal preparation.
- Can be challenging to follow when eating out or in social situations.
- Switching to low-sodium foods may take time to adjust to the change in taste.

## 7-Day Meal Plan

Note: Be sure to consult a healthcare professional before starting this or any other meal plan. Portion sizes and food variety may vary based on individual needs.

Day 1
- Breakfast: Oatmeal with mixed berries and nuts.
- Lunch: Tuna salad with lettuce, tomato, cucumber, and olive oil and balsamic vinegar dressing.
- Dinner: Grilled chicken breast with green salad and baked potatoes.
- Snack: Greek yogurt with mixed berries.

Day 2
- Breakfast: Whole wheat toast with avocado and poached egg.
- Lunch: Vegetable soup with a handful of lentils.

- Dinner: Baked salmon with steamed broccoli and quinoa.
- Snack: Apple with almond butter.

Day 3
- Breakfast: Spinach, banana, and almond butter smoothie.
- Lunch: Chickpea salad with spinach, cucumber, tomato, and tahini dressing.
- Dinner: Baked white fish with quinoa and roasted vegetables.
- Snack: Carrots and hummus.

Day 4
- Breakfast: Whole grain cereal with skim milk and mixed berries.
- Lunch: Chicken salad with lettuce, tomato, carrot, and low-sodium dressing.
- Dinner: Baked hake fillet with roasted potatoes and steamed broccoli.
- Snack: Greek yogurt with nuts.

Day 5
- Breakfast: Egg white omelet with spinach and mushrooms.
- Lunch: Lentil salad with raw vegetables and olive oil and balsamic vinegar dressing.
- Dinner: Grilled chicken breast with green salad and quinoa.
- Snack: Apple with almond butter.

Day 6
- Breakfast: Protein smoothie with banana, spinach, and almond butter.
- Lunch: Tuna salad with lettuce, tomato, cucumber, and olive oil and balsamic vinegar dressing.
- Dinner: Baked salmon with quinoa and steamed asparagus.
- Snack: Carrots and hummus.

Day 7
- Breakfast: Whole wheat toast with avocado and poached egg.
- Lunch: Lentil soup with vegetables and a slice of whole grain bread.
- Dinner: Grilled white fish with mixed salad and baked sweet

potato.
- Snack: Greek yogurt with mixed berries.

The DASH Diet can be a suitable option for individuals looking to improve their cardiovascular health and maintain overall well-being. However, it's important to remember that each individual is different, and what works for one person may not work for another. It's always recommended to consult with a healthcare professional before making significant changes to your diet.

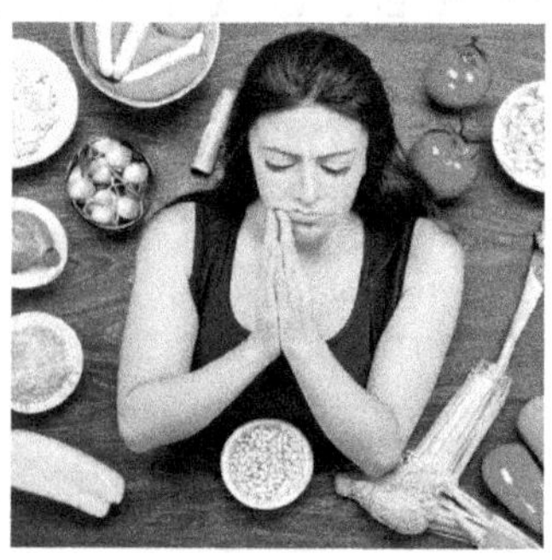

## Chapter 9: Portion Control Diet

Introduction to the Portion Control Diet

The Portion Control Diet doesn't focus as much on what foods you should eat but rather on how much you should eat. It's an approach that takes into account the number of calories consumed and aims to balance the energy taken into the body with the energy expended. The primary goal is to help individuals better understand appropriate food portions and avoid overeating.

Benefits and Challenges

Benefits:
- Can aid in weight loss and prevent weight gain.
- Provides greater flexibility regarding the types of foods that can

be eaten.
- Can help increase awareness of the body's nutritional and energy needs.

Challenges:
- Requires consistent and mindful tracking of the amount of food consumed.
- Can be challenging to follow when eating out or in social situations.
- Takes time to learn and understand appropriate portions of different types of foods.

7-Day Meal Plan

Note: Be sure to consult a healthcare professional before starting this or any other meal plan. Portion sizes and food variety may vary based on individual needs.

Day 1
- Breakfast: Oatmeal (1/2 cup) with mixed berries (1 cup) and nuts (1/4 cup).
- Lunch: Chicken salad (1 cup chicken, 2 cups mixed vegetables).
- Dinner: Grilled salmon fillet (100g), steamed asparagus (1 cup), and baked potatoes (1/2 medium potato).
- Snack: Apple (1 medium) with almond butter (1 tablespoon).

Day 2
- Breakfast: Whole wheat toast (1 slice) with avocado (1/2 avocado) and poached egg (1 egg).
- Lunch: Vegetable soup (1 cup) with a handful of chickpeas (1/2 cup).
- Dinner: Grilled chicken breast (100g), green salad (2 cups), and quinoa (1/2 cup).
- Snack: Greek yogurt (1 cup) with mixed berries (1/2 cup).

Day 3
- Breakfast: Spinach (1 cup), banana (1/2 banana), and almond butter (1 tablespoon) smoothie.

- Lunch: Tuna salad (1 can), lettuce (2 cups), tomato (1 medium tomato), and cucumber (1/2 cucumber).
- Dinner: Baked white fish (100g), quinoa (1/2 cup), and roasted vegetables (1 cup).
- Snack: Carrots (1 cup) and hummus (2 tablespoons).

This day provides a variety of nutrients through balanced and healthy meals. As with any diet, it's important to pay attention to hunger and satiety cues to adjust portions as needed.

Day 4
- Breakfast: Whole grain cereal (1 cup) with skim milk (1 cup) and mixed berries (1/2 cup).
- Lunch: Quinoa salad (1/2 cup quinoa, 1 cup mixed vegetables) with grilled chicken (100g).
- Dinner: Baked hake fillet (100g) with roasted potatoes (1/2 medium potato) and steamed broccoli (1 cup).
- Snack: Greek yogurt (1 cup) with nuts (1/4 cup).

Day 5
- Breakfast: Egg white omelet (2 egg whites) with spinach (1 cup) and mushrooms (1/2 cup).
- Lunch: Lentil salad (1/2 cup lentils, 2 cups raw vegetables) with olive oil (1 tablespoon) and balsamic vinegar (1 tablespoon) dressing.
- Dinner: Grilled chicken breast (100g) with green salad (2 cups) and baked sweet potato (1/2 medium potato).
- Snack: Apple (1 medium) with almond butter (1 tablespoon).

Day 6
- Breakfast: Protein shake (1 scoop) with banana (1/2 banana), spinach (1 cup), and almond butter (1 tablespoon).
- Lunch: Chicken salad (1 cup chicken, 2 cups mixed vegetables).
- Dinner: Baked salmon (100g) with quinoa (1/2 cup) and steamed asparagus (1 cup).
- Snack: Carrots (1 cup) and hummus (2 tablespoons).

Day 7

- Breakfast: Whole wheat toast (1 slice) with avocado (1/2 avocado) and poached egg (1 egg).
- Lunch: Lentil soup (1 cup) with vegetables (1 cup) and a slice of whole grain bread (1 slice).
- Dinner: Grilled white fish (100g) with mixed salad (2 cups) and baked potato (1/2 medium potato).
- Snack: Greek yogurt (1 cup) with mixed berries (1/2 cup).

The Portion Control Diet can be an excellent option for individuals who want to lose weight and improve their overall health. However, it's important to remember that everyone is different, and what works for one person may not work for another. It's always advisable to consult with a healthcare professional before making significant changes to your diet.

## Chapter 10: Low-Carb Diet

Introduction to the Low-Carb Diet

The Low-Carb Diet focuses on reducing carbohydrate intake and, in many cases, increasing the consumption of protein and healthy fats. This diet has gained popularity due to its effectiveness in weight loss and blood sugar control. Typical foods in this diet include meats, fish, eggs, vegetables, fruits, nuts, and seeds.

Benefits and Challenges
Benefits:
• Can promote weight loss.
• Can help control blood sugar levels.
• Can improve cardiovascular health by reducing triglyceride levels.

Challenges:
• Limiting carbohydrate intake can be difficult, especially at the beginning.
• May cause temporary side effects such as fatigue, headache, and constipation.
• It is challenging to follow when eating out or in social events.

7-Day Meal Plan
Note: Make sure to consult with a healthcare professional before starting this or any other meal plan. Portion sizes and food variety may vary based on individual needs.

Day 1
- Breakfast: Spinach and feta cheese omelette with avocado.
- Lunch: Chicken salad with olive oil dressing.
- Dinner: Grilled salmon with asparagus.
- Snack: Almonds and cottage cheese.

Day 2
- Breakfast: Protein shake with almond butter and berries.
- Lunch: Tuna salad with olives and cucumber.
- Dinner: Baked chicken with steamed broccoli.
- Snack: Greek yogurt with nuts.

Day 3
- Breakfast: Egg and cheese omelette with tomatoes.
- Lunch: Shrimp salad with olive oil dressing.
- Dinner: Grilled red meat (beef) steak with green salad.
- Snack: Celery with almond butter.

Day 4
- Breakfast: Protein shake with almond butter and chia seeds.
- Lunch: Chicken salad with avocado and walnuts.
- Dinner: Baked salmon with spinach salad.
- Snack: Cheese and olives.

Day 5
- Breakfast: Scrambled eggs with mushrooms and cheddar cheese.
- Lunch: Tuna salad with olive oil dressing.
- Dinner: Grilled chicken breast with broccoli.
- Snack: Greek yogurt with flax seeds.

Day 6
- Breakfast: Spinach and feta cheese omelette.
- Lunch: Chicken salad with olive oil dressing.

- Dinner: Grilled beef steak with green salad.
- Snack: Almonds and cottage cheese.

Day 7
- Breakfast: Protein shake with almond butter and berries.
- Lunch: Shrimp salad with olive oil dressing.
- Dinner: Grilled salmon with steamed asparagus.
- Snack: Celery with almond butter.

Remember, although this diet plan can help promote weight loss, it's important to follow a balanced diet that includes a variety of foods to ensure you're getting essential nutrients. It's always best to consult with a healthcare professional before starting a new diet or meal plan.

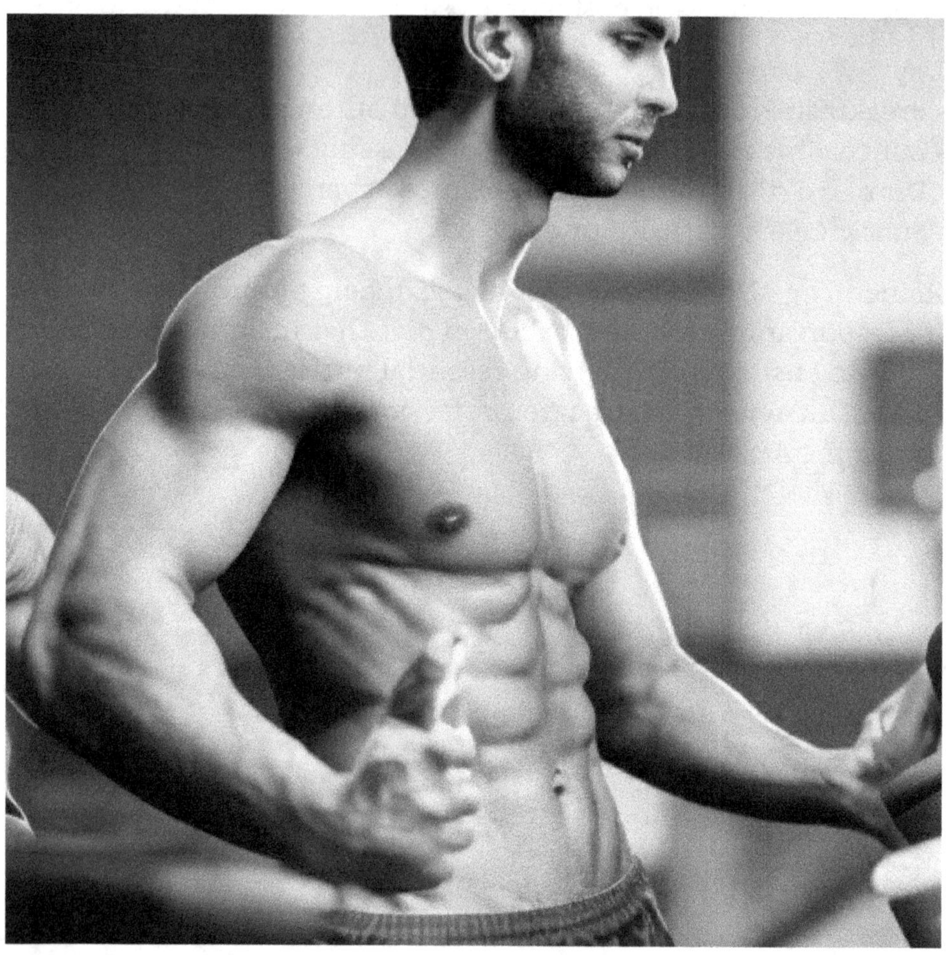

## Conclusion

We have embarked on an interesting and educational journey through various diets that have proven beneficial for weight loss. However, it is important to remember that each body is unique, and what works for one person may not work for another.

Choosing the Right Diet for You
When choosing the right diet, it is important to consider several factors. First, consider your health and wellness goals. Are you looking to lose weight, improve cardiovascular health, manage a chronic condition like diabetes, or simply adopt healthier eating habits?

Additionally, it's important to consider your preferences and lifestyle. If you don't like meat, for example, a plant-based diet plan may be a good option for you. If you have a busy schedule and limited time for cooking, a diet that includes pre-made or easy-to-prepare meals may be more suitable.

Finally, it is crucial to remember that any diet you choose should be sustainable in the long term. It makes no sense to adopt an extremely restrictive diet that you cannot maintain. The best diet is one that you can follow in the long run, that fits your tastes and lifestyle, and that helps you achieve your health goals.

Maintaining Long-Term Changes
Losing weight is not simply a matter of following a short-term diet, but of making lasting changes in your eating habits and lifestyle. To maintain the weight loss, it is important to follow a proper diet and engage in physical activity.

Furthermore, it is essential to learn how to manage stress and take care of your mental health. Many times, people turn to food as a way of coping with stress or negative emotions. Learning stress management techniques and taking care of your emotional well-being can be just as important as taking care of your physical health.

**Additional Resources**

There are numerous resources available to assist you on your journey to a healthier life. This includes registered dietitians, health and wellness coaches, weight loss support groups, and a wide variety of books, websites, and mobile apps dedicated to nutrition and weight loss.

Additionally, don't forget the resources included in this book, such as additional recipes, a glossary of terms, and references for further reading. These can be valuable tools to assist you on your path to a healthier and happier life.

In conclusion, the journey to weight loss and a healthier life is just that—a journey. It's not about perfection but about making small sustainable changes that add up to significant results over time. We wish you success on your journey.

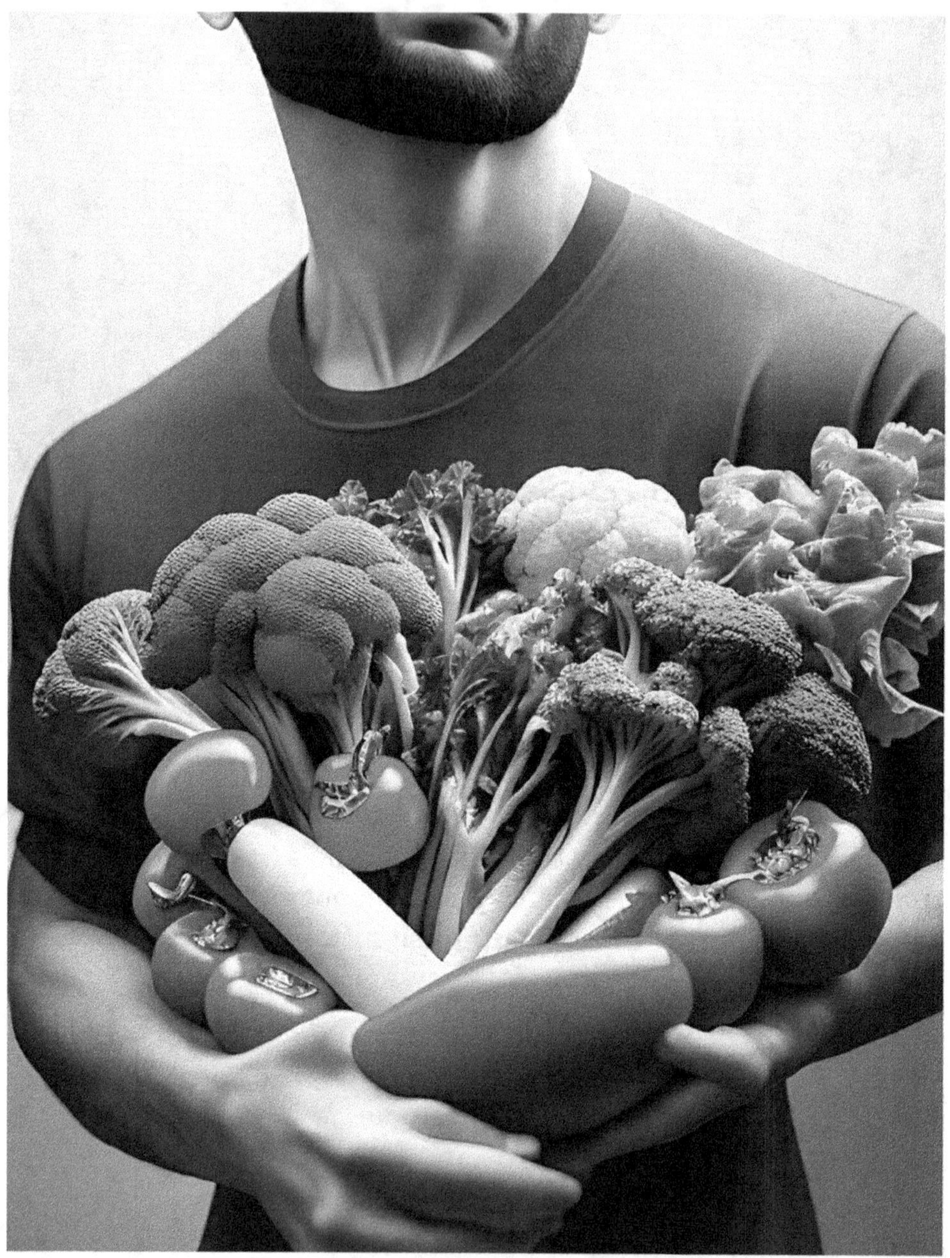

## Appendix
This book has made an effort to provide a detailed and easily

understandable analysis of various effective weight loss diet plans. However, we understand that some terms and concepts may be new to some readers. That's why we have included this appendix to provide further information and clarify any confusion.

Glossary of Terms
• Lean proteins: Protein sources that contain less fat. Examples: chicken breast, fish, tofu.
• Complex carbohydrates: Carbohydrates that break down slowly in the body, providing sustained energy. Examples: oatmeal, brown rice, quinoa.
• Fiber: A nutrient that aids digestion and can help with weight control. Found in foods such as fruits, vegetables, legumes, and whole grains.
• Healthy fats: Fats that are beneficial for heart health. Examples: avocados, nuts, seeds, fatty fish.

Additional Recipes
Here are some additional recipes for each diet plan:
Mediterranean Diet
• Roasted Vegetable Quinoa Salad: Cooked quinoa, roasted vegetables (such as peppers, zucchini, and eggplant), dressed with olive oil, lemon juice, salt, and pepper.

Whole Foods Plant-Based Diet
• Red Lentil Curry: Red lentils, onion, garlic, ginger, tomato, cumin, turmeric, cilantro, and coconut milk.

Lean Proteins and Veget ables Diet
• Chicken and Broccoli Stir-Fry: Chicken breast, broccoli, garlic, low-sodium soy sauce, ginger, and sesame oil.

Low-Carb Diet
• Zucchini Noodles with Meatballs: Zucchini, lean ground beef, garlic, tomato, oregano, and olive oil.

## References and Further Reading

This book has been informed by a variety of scientific and nutrition expert sources. Here are some references and further reading for those who wish to learn more:

1. Ludwig, D. S. (2018). Always Hungry?: Conquer Cravings, Retrain Your Fat Cells, and Lose Weight Permanently. Hachette Books.
2. Willett, W., & Skerrett, P. J. (2017). Eat, Drink, and Be Healthy: The Harvard Medical School Guide to Healthy Eating. Free Press.
3. Ornish, D. (2007). The Spectrum: A Scientifically Proven Program to Feel Better, Live Longer, Lose Weight, and Gain Health. Ballantine Books.
4. Fung, J. (2016). The Obesity Code: Unlocking the Secrets of Weight Loss. Greystone Books.
5. Mosley, M. (2018). The Clever Guts Diet: How to Revolutionize Your Body from the Inside Out. Atria Books.
6. Davis, W. (2014). Wheat Belly: Lose the Wheat, Lose the Weight, and Find Your Path Back to Health. Rodale Books.

In addition to printed resources, there are many online websites and blogs that provide additional information and support for weight loss and healthy eating. Here are some suggestions:

• www.nutritionfacts.org: A nonprofit website that provides evidence-based information on nutrition and health.
• www.eatright.org: The website of the Academy of Nutrition and Dietetics offers a variety of resources on nutrition and wellness.

• www.cdc.gov/healthyweight: The website of the Centers for Disease Control and Prevention (CDC) provides resources on maintaining a healthy weight.
• www.heart.org: The American Heart Association has a section dedicated to healthy eating and weight loss.
• www.hsph.harvard.edu/nutritionsource: Harvard School of Public Health offers evidence-based information on nutrition.

We hope that these additional resources and references provided are useful to you on your journey toward a healthier and happier life. Remember, the journey is yours, and every small change you make can have a significant impact on your long-term health and well-being. Good luck on your journey to a healthier life!